The Simple Weight Loss Guide

Daniel Payne

DEDICATION

This book is dedicated to all those who work hard for what they want and celebrate each achievement, no matter how small, along the way.

CONTENTS

ACKNOWLEDGMENTS

All of the information herein is common sense. There is no revolutionary way to lose weight and keep it off, but there are certain ways to lose weight and keep it off. You will find those techniques in this book. Acknowledgement is given to those who know that shortcuts hardly ever work and that nothing worthwhile is easy.

1 Introduction

Losing weight and maintaining a healthy weight is a multifaceted process that involves a combination of lifestyle changes and behavioral modifications. Here are the top 10 ways to achieve weight loss and keep it off in the long term:

Set Realistic Goals: Start by setting achievable and realistic weight loss goals. Aim for steady and gradual weight loss, typically around 1-2 pounds per week. Unrealistic expectations can lead to disappointment and give up on your weight loss journey.

Create a Calorie Deficit: Weight loss primarily occurs when you consume fewer calories than your body burns for energy. This can be achieved by a combination of eating fewer calories and increasing physical activity. Calculate your basal metabolic rate (BMR) and daily calorie needs to establish a healthy caloric deficit.

Adopt a Balanced Diet: Focus on a balanced diet that includes a variety of nutrient-dense foods such as fruits, vegetables, lean proteins, whole grains, and healthy fats. Minimize the intake of processed foods, sugary beverages, and high-calorie snacks. A balanced diet ensures you get all the essential nutrients while losing weight.

Practice Portion Control: Pay attention to portion sizes to avoid overeating. Use smaller plates and bowls to help control your food intake visually. Mindful eating techniques, such as eating slowly and savoring each bite, can also prevent overeating.

Regular Physical Activity: Incorporate regular exercise into your routine. Aim for at least 150 minutes of moderate-intensity aerobic activity or 75 minutes of vigorous-intensity aerobic activity per week, along with muscle-strengthening activities on two or more days per week. Find physical activities you enjoy to make it sustainable.

Stay Hydrated: Drink plenty of water throughout the day. Sometimes, thirst can be mistaken for hunger, leading to unnecessary calorie consumption. Water can also help you feel fuller, reducing the urge to overeat.

Get Enough Sleep: Quality sleep is essential for weight management. Lack of sleep can disrupt hunger hormones and lead to weight gain. Aim for 7-9 hours of sleep per night to support your weight loss efforts.

Manage Stress: Chronic stress can lead to emotional eating and hinder weight loss progress. Find healthy ways to manage stress, such as meditation, yoga, deep breathing exercises, or engaging in hobbies you enjoy.

Track Your Progress: Keep a food journal or use a mobile app to track your food intake, exercise, and weight loss progress. Monitoring your behaviors and achievements can help you stay accountable and identify areas for improvement.

Build a Support System: Surround yourself with a supportive network of friends, family, or even a weight loss group. Having a support system can provide encouragement, motivation, and accountability throughout your weight loss journey.

Remember that sustainable weight loss takes time and dedication. It's essential to focus on developing healthy habits rather than quick fixes or fad diets. Gradual progress and consistency are key to achieving and maintaining a healthy weight in the long term. If you have any underlying health conditions or concerns, it's best to consult with a healthcare professional or registered dietitian before starting any weight loss program.

2 Setting Realistic Goals

Setting realistic goals is a crucial step in achieving successful and sustainable weight loss. Often, individuals embark on weight loss journeys with grandiose expectations, only to become discouraged when they don't see immediate results. In this chapter, we will explore the importance of setting achievable and realistic goals, understanding the psychology behind goal-setting, and practical strategies for establishing targets that pave the way for long-term weight loss success.

Understanding the Psychology of Goal-Setting

Human behavior is profoundly influenced by goal-setting, and it plays a significant role in weight loss efforts. However, not all goals are created equal. Unrealistic or overly ambitious goals can lead to frustration and disappointment, while setting attainable milestones boosts motivation and fosters a sense of accomplishment.

Specificity: Vague goals such as "losing weight" can be overwhelming and lack direction. Instead, set specific objectives like "losing 1-2 pounds per week" or "reducing waist circumference by 2 inches." Specific goals provide clarity and a roadmap to follow.

Measurability: Ensure that your goals are measurable. Being able to track progress allows you to celebrate achievements and make necessary adjustments to your weight loss plan. For instance, "eating five servings of vegetables daily" is measurable, while "eating more veggies" is not.
Attainability: Aim for goals that are within your reach. Setting impossible targets may lead to a sense of failure. Consider your current lifestyle, commitments, and resources when determining what is achievable.

Relevance: Your weight loss goals should align with your overall health and well-being objectives. Focus on the reasons why you want to lose weight, such as improving your energy levels, reducing the risk of chronic diseases, or enhancing self-confidence.

Time-Bound: Set a timeframe for achieving your weight loss goals. This prevents procrastination and provides a sense of urgency to stay on track. For example, "losing 15 pounds in three months" sets a clear deadline.

The Power of Small Steps

Breaking down larger weight loss goals into smaller, manageable steps can be a game-changer. Smaller milestones are less overwhelming and provide a sense of accomplishment more frequently. It's essential to celebrate each achievement, no matter how modest, as it reinforces positive behavior and encourages continued progress.

Setting short-term goals, such as adopting healthier eating habits or increasing daily physical activity, can lead to significant long-term results. These small successes create a positive feedback loop, enhancing your motivation to persevere.

The SMART Approach to Goal-Setting

The SMART approach is a widely used method for setting realistic and achievable goals. It stands for Specific, Measurable, Achievable, Relevant, and Time-Bound. Applying the SMART criteria to weight loss goals can significantly improve your chances of success.

> Specific: Define your weight loss goal with precision. Instead of saying, "I want to lose weight," specify the amount of weight you want to lose and how you plan to do it.

Measurable: Establish how you will track your progress. This could be through regular weigh-ins, body measurements, or monitoring dietary and exercise habits.

Achievable: Ensure your goal is realistic and attainable based on your current circumstances, such as work schedule, family commitments, and existing health conditions.

Relevant: Consider why this goal matters to you and how it aligns with your values and long-term aspirations for a healthier lifestyle. Time-Bound: Set a deadline for reaching your weight loss goal. This creates a sense of urgency and provides a timeframe for evaluating progress and making adjustments.

Flexibility and Adaptability

It's essential to recognize that life is dynamic, and circumstances may change as you progress on your weight loss journey. Be prepared to adjust your goals as needed and avoid being too rigid. Embrace flexibility and view setbacks as opportunities to learn and grow.

Maintaining a positive attitude and a growth mindset are crucial elements in sustaining motivation throughout your weight loss journey. Be kind to yourself and acknowledge that progress may not always be linear.

Conclusion

Setting realistic goals for weight loss is a fundamental step in achieving success on your journey toward a healthier lifestyle. By applying the principles of specificity, measurability, attainability, relevance, and time-bound targets, you create a solid foundation for lasting change.

Embrace the power of small steps, celebrate your achievements, and be willing to adapt as needed. Remember that weight loss is a gradual process that requires patience, perseverance, and a commitment to self-improvement. By setting realistic goals and staying focused on the bigger picture, you can achieve and maintain your desired weight while experiencing improved overall well-being and increased confidence in yourself and your abilities

3 Creating a Calorie Deficit

Creating a calorie deficit is the cornerstone of successful weight loss. At its core, weight loss occurs when you consume fewer calories than your body expends. In this chapter, we will delve into the concept of calorie deficit, understand its significance in weight loss, explore various methods to achieve it, and provide practical tips to ensure a healthy and sustainable approach to shedding unwanted pounds.

Understanding the Calorie Deficit

A calorie deficit is the energy gap between the number of calories you consume through food and beverages and the number of calories your body burns through metabolism and physical activity. When you maintain a calorie deficit over time, your body turns to stored fat for energy, leading to weight loss.

> Calories In vs. Calories Out: The principle of "calories in vs. calories out" lies at the heart of weight management. To lose weight, you must consume fewer calories than your body burns. Conversely, to gain weight, you need to consume more calories than your body expends.

BMR and TDEE: Your Basal Metabolic Rate (BMR) represents the number of calories your body needs to maintain basic physiological functions at rest. Total Daily Energy Expenditure (TDEE) includes BMR plus calories burned through physical activity. To create a calorie deficit, you can either decrease your caloric intake, increase your physical activity, or combine both strategies.

Methods to Create a Calorie Deficit

Dietary Modifications: Adopting a balanced and mindful approach to eating can help you create a calorie deficit without feeling deprived.

- Portion Control: Pay attention to portion sizes to avoid overeating. Use smaller plates and bowls to manage portions visually.
- Caloric Density: Choose foods that are lower in caloric density, such as fruits and vegetables, which can help you feel full with fewer calories.
- Meal Planning: Plan your meals in advance to ensure that you make healthier choices and avoid impulsive, high-calorie options.

- Tracking Food Intake: Keep a food journal or use a mobile app to log your meals and snacks. This practice can help you become more aware of your eating habits and identify areas for improvement.
- Mindful Eating: Slow down and savor each bite, paying attention to hunger and satiety cues. This approach can prevent overeating and promote a healthier relationship with food.

Regular Exercise: Physical activity not only contributes to a calorie deficit but also offers numerous health benefits.

- Aerobic Exercise: Engage in activities such as walking, jogging, cycling, or swimming to burn calories and increase your overall energy expenditure.
- Strength Training: Incorporate resistance training to build lean muscle mass, which can boost your metabolism and help you burn more calories at rest.
- Interval Training: High-Intensity Interval Training (HIIT) alternates short bursts of intense exercise with brief recovery periods, effectively burning more calories in a shorter time.

- Non-Exercise Activity: Increase your daily activity levels by taking the stairs, walking during breaks, or incorporating physical activity into your daily routine.

Tips for a Healthy and Sustainable Calorie Deficit

Avoid Extreme Diets: Very low-calorie diets or crash diets can lead to nutrient deficiencies, muscle loss, and a slowed metabolism. Instead, focus on a balanced and varied diet that provides all essential nutrients.

Gradual Progress: Aim for a moderate calorie deficit rather than drastic cuts. This approach is more sustainable and helps preserve lean muscle mass.

Stay Hydrated: Drink plenty of water throughout the day. Sometimes, thirst can be mistaken for hunger, leading to unnecessary calorie consumption.

Monitor Progress: Keep track of your weight loss and adjust your caloric intake and activity levels as needed. Consistent monitoring allows you to fine-tune your approach and stay on track.

Seek Professional Guidance: If you are unsure about creating a calorie deficit or have underlying health conditions, consult with a registered dietitian or healthcare professional to develop a personalized weight loss plan.

Conclusion

Creating a calorie deficit is a fundamental component of successful weight loss. By understanding the concept of "calories in vs. calories out" and implementing dietary modifications and regular physical activity, you can achieve a healthy and sustainable calorie deficit. Embrace a balanced and mindful approach to eating, stay consistent with your exercise routine, and remember that gradual progress is the key to achieving and maintaining your weight loss goals. With patience, dedication, and a focus on overall well-being, you can embark on a rewarding journey toward a healthier and happier you.

4 A Balanced Diet

Adopting a balanced diet is a cornerstone of maintaining optimal health and achieving sustainable weight loss. A balanced diet provides the body with essential nutrients, energy, and a diverse range of foods that support overall well-being. In this chapter, we will explore the components of a balanced diet, understand the importance of nutrient variety, and provide practical tips to help you adapt and embrace a balanced eating pattern.

Components of a Balanced Diet

A balanced diet comprises a mix of nutrients that fulfill the body's needs for growth, energy, and maintenance. The key components include:

Fruits and Vegetables: These are rich in vitamins, minerals, fiber, and antioxidants. Aim to fill half your plate with colorful fruits and vegetables to support immune function, digestion, and overall health.

Proteins: Include lean protein sources such as poultry, fish, lean meats, legumes, nuts, seeds, and low-fat dairy. Protein is essential for muscle repair, immune function, and hormone production.

Whole Grains: Opt for whole grains like brown rice, quinoa, whole wheat, and oats. They provide complex carbohydrates for sustained energy and fiber that aids digestion and promotes a feeling of fullness.

Healthy Fats: Incorporate sources of unsaturated fats, including avocados, nuts, seeds, and olive oil. These fats support heart health, brain function, and nutrient absorption.

Dairy or Dairy Alternatives: Choose low-fat or non-fat dairy products or fortified plant-based alternatives for calcium, vitamin D, and other essential nutrients.

Moderation and Portion Control: While no food is off-limits, practice moderation and portion control for foods higher in added sugars, saturated fats, and sodium.

Importance of Nutrient Variety

Nutrient Density: A variety of nutrient-dense foods ensures you obtain essential vitamins, minerals, and antioxidants without excess calories. Nutrient density is a key factor in achieving satiety and overall well-being.

Micronutrient Balance: Different foods contain different micronutrients. A diverse diet helps prevent deficiencies and ensures you receive a broad spectrum of nutrients required for bodily functions.

Diverse Gut Microbiota: Consuming a range of foods promotes a diverse gut microbiota, which contributes to digestion, immune function, and overall health.

Sustainability: A diverse diet is more sustainable, as it prevents monotony and encourages enjoyment of a wide array of flavors and textures.

Practical Tips for Adapting a Balanced Diet

Plan Meals: Design a weekly meal plan that incorporates a variety of foods from all food groups. This helps you make healthier choices and reduces the likelihood of reaching for convenience foods.

Experiment with New Foods: Explore new fruits, vegetables, grains, and protein sources.

Trying different foods can be a fun way to expand your palate and nutrient intake.

Use the "Plate Method": Divide your plate into quarters. Fill one-half with vegetables, one-quarter with lean protein, and one-quarter with whole grains or starchy vegetables.

Choose Colorful Foods: Vibrantly colored foods often signify a high content of vitamins and antioxidants. Aim for a colorful plate to ensure nutrient variety.

Read Labels: Pay attention to food labels to make informed choices about nutrient content, serving sizes, and added sugars or unhealthy fats.

Hydration: Include plenty of water in your diet. Staying hydrated supports digestion, metabolism, and overall vitality.

Listen to Hunger and Fullness Cues: Eat mindfully, paying attention to when you are hungry and when you are comfortably full. Avoid overeating and respect your body's signals.

Conclusion

Adapting a balanced diet is essential for promoting overall health, maintaining a healthy weight, and preventing chronic diseases. By including a variety of nutrient-dense foods from all food groups, you provide your body with the essential building blocks it needs to function optimally. Remember that balance is key—enjoy a wide range of foods in moderation while being mindful of portion sizes. By making informed choices, experimenting with new foods, and embracing nutrient variety, you can create a sustainable eating pattern that supports your lifelong wellness journey.

5 Portion Control

Practicing portion control is a fundamental strategy for achieving weight loss goals and maintaining a healthy lifestyle. It involves consuming the right amount of food to meet your body's needs while avoiding overindulgence. In this chapter, we will delve into the importance of portion control, understand its impact on weight management, explore practical techniques for portion control, and provide tips to help you develop mindful eating habits.

The Significance of Portion Control

Portion control plays a pivotal role in weight management by helping you regulate calorie intake and maintain a healthy balance between the calories you consume and the calories you burn. In a culture where larger portions are prevalent, practicing portion control can prevent overeating and contribute to successful weight loss.

Caloric Intake Regulation: By managing portion sizes, you can regulate your caloric intake and create a calorie deficit, which is essential for weight loss.

Mindful Eating: Portion control encourages mindful eating, where you pay attention to your body's hunger and fullness cues, making it easier to recognize when you're satisfied.

Prevention of Overeating: Oversized portions can lead to consuming excess calories, which ultimately hinder weight loss efforts and contribute to weight gain.

Practical Techniques for Portion Control

Use Visual Cues:
- Use your hand as a guide: For example, a portion of lean protein is roughly the size of your palm, while a serving of grains fits within your closed fist.
- Divide your plate: Use the plate method, allocating a portion for protein, vegetables, and whole grains. Aim for half the plate to be filled with non-starchy vegetables.

Measure and Weigh:
- Invest in a kitchen scale and measuring cups to accurately measure portions of food.

- Read nutrition labels to identify serving sizes and compare them to what you're actually consuming.

Choose Smaller Plates and Bowls:

- Opt for smaller dinnerware to visually control portion sizes. A smaller plate can create the illusion of a more substantial meal.

Avoid Eating from Containers:

- Serve your food onto a plate instead of eating directly from bags or containers. This prevents mindless overeating.

Restaurant Strategies:

- Share meals or order appetizer-sized portions at restaurants.
- Ask for dressings, sauces, and condiments on the side to control how much you use.

Developing Mindful Eating Habits

Eat Slowly:

- Take your time to savor each bite. Eating slowly allows your body to register fullness and prevents overeating.

Pay Attention to Hunger and Fullness:

- Before eating, assess your hunger level on a scale of 1 to 10. Aim to start eating when you're moderately hungry and stop when you're comfortably satisfied.

Practice the "Three Bite Rule":

- Take three bites of a treat or indulgent food to satisfy your craving, then put it away. Often, the first few bites provide the most enjoyment.

Pause During Meals:

- Put down your utensils between bites and take a moment to check in with your body. This helps you gauge if you need more food or if you're content.

Conclusion

Practicing portion control is an integral aspect of achieving and maintaining weight loss goals. By becoming mindful of portion sizes, you can regulate your calorie intake, prevent overeating, and create a sustainable eating pattern that supports long-term weight management. Incorporate visual cues, measuring tools, and mindful eating techniques into your routine to develop a healthier relationship with food and gain control over your eating habits. Remember that portion control is not about deprivation but about making informed choices and enjoying food in a balanced and mindful manner.

6 REGULAR PHYSICAL ACTIVITY

Regular physical activity is a vital component of a successful weight loss journey and overall well-being. It not only aids in creating a calorie deficit but also offers a plethora of health benefits that contribute to improved fitness, mental health, and quality of life. In this chapter, we will delve into the significance of incorporating regular physical activity into your routine, explore its role in weight loss, discuss various types of exercises, and provide practical strategies to make exercise an enjoyable and sustainable part of your life.

The Role of Physical Activity in Weight Loss

Physical activity is a key factor in achieving and maintaining weight loss for several reasons:

Calorie Expenditure: Engaging in physical activity burns calories, contributing to the calorie deficit required for weight loss.

Metabolism Boost: Regular exercise can increase your metabolism, helping your body burn more calories even at rest.

Preservation of Lean Muscle: Exercise, particularly strength training, helps preserve lean muscle mass while losing weight. More muscle mass increases the body's calorie-burning potential.

Appetite Regulation: Physical activity can help regulate appetite hormones, potentially reducing cravings and overeating.

Enhanced Fat Loss: Certain types of exercises, like high-intensity interval training (HIIT), can promote fat loss and improve body composition.

Types of Physical Activities for Weight Loss

Aerobic Exercises:
- Activities like brisk walking, jogging, cycling, swimming, and dancing increase heart rate and contribute to calorie burning.
- Aim for at least 150 minutes of moderate-intensity aerobic activity or 75 minutes of vigorous-intensity aerobic activity per week.

Strength Training:
- Lifting weights or using resistance bands builds muscle and increases metabolism.

- Include strength training exercises for major muscle groups on two or more days per week.

High-Intensity Interval Training (HIIT):

- HIIT alternates between short bursts of intense activity and periods of rest or low-intensity exercise.
- HIIT can burn a significant amount of calories in a shorter time, making it efficient for weight loss.

Flexibility and Balance Exercises:

- Activities like yoga and Pilates improve flexibility, balance, and overall body awareness.

Practical Strategies to Make Physical Activity a Habit

Find Activities You Enjoy:

- Engage in activities that you find enjoyable, whether it's dancing, hiking, swimming, or playing a sport. This increases the likelihood of sticking with it.

Set Realistic Goals:

- Establish achievable fitness goals, such as walking a certain number of steps each day or increasing your workout intensity gradually.

Incorporate Movement into Your Day:

- Use active transportation, take the stairs, and stand or walk during phone calls to increase daily activity levels.

Create a Routine:

- Schedule regular exercise sessions into your week, treating them as non-negotiable appointments.

Buddy System:

- Exercise with a friend or join a group fitness class to stay motivated and accountable.

Track Your Progress:

- Keep a workout journal or use fitness apps to track your exercises, monitor improvements, and celebrate milestones.

Conclusion

Regular physical activity is a cornerstone of successful weight loss and overall well-being. By incorporating various types of exercises into your routine, you can create a calorie deficit, boost metabolism, and preserve lean muscle mass. Remember that exercise is not only about weight loss—it's a powerful tool that enhances your physical and mental health, increases energy levels, and promotes longevity. By finding activities you enjoy, setting achievable goals, and making physical activity a habit, you can embark on a fulfilling fitness journey that supports your weight loss goals and leads to a healthier, happier you.

7 Staying Hydrated

Staying hydrated is a foundational element of overall health and a key factor in successful weight loss. Water is essential for numerous bodily functions, including metabolism, digestion, and energy production. In this chapter, we will explore the importance of hydration for weight loss, understand how water influences the body's processes, discuss the role of hydration in appetite regulation, and provide practical tips to ensure you stay adequately hydrated on your weight loss journey.

The Link Between Hydration and Weight Loss

Metabolism Boost: Proper hydration supports efficient metabolic processes. Studies suggest that adequate hydration can temporarily boost metabolic rate, aiding in calorie burning. Digestion and Nutrient Absorption: Water helps break down food and aids in the absorption of nutrients. Efficient digestion contributes to overall well-being and can positively impact weight loss efforts.

Appetite Suppression: Staying hydrated can help curb appetite and prevent overeating.

Sometimes, thirst is mistaken for hunger, leading to unnecessary calorie consumption.

Fluid Balance: Adequate hydration supports fluid balance in cells, tissues, and organs, optimizing bodily functions and promoting overall health.

Hydration and Appetite Regulation

Thirst and Hunger Connection: The brain's thirst and hunger centers are closely connected. Staying hydrated can help prevent overeating by reducing the chances of confusing thirst with hunger.

Satiety Signal: Drinking water before or during meals can enhance feelings of fullness, potentially leading to reduced food intake.

Optimal Digestion: Hydration supports smooth digestion, preventing digestive discomfort that might lead to overeating or unhealthy food choices.

Practical Tips for Staying Hydrated

Monitor Fluid Intake:
- Aim to drink at least 8 glasses (about 2 liters) of water per day. Your actual

needs may vary based on factors such as climate, activity level, and individual differences.

Hydrate Throughout the Day:

- Sip water consistently throughout the day rather than consuming large amounts at once. This helps maintain steady hydration levels.

Incorporate Hydrating Foods:

- Consume water-rich foods like fruits (e.g., watermelon, oranges) and vegetables (e.g., cucumber, lettuce) to contribute to your daily hydration.

Listen to Your Body:

- Pay attention to thirst cues and drink when you feel thirsty. Additionally, observe the color of your urine—pale yellow indicates proper hydration.

Hydrate Before Meals:

- Drink a glass of water before meals to support digestion and help regulate appetite.

Stay Hydrated During Exercise:

- Drink water before, during, and after exercise to replace fluids lost through sweat and support optimal performance.

Limit Sugary Beverages:

- Minimize consumption of sugary beverages like sodas and fruit juices.

These can contribute to excess calorie intake without providing essential nutrients.

Conclusion

Staying hydrated is a fundamental aspect of successful weight loss and overall well-being. Proper hydration supports metabolism, digestion, appetite regulation, and fluid balance. By incorporating practical hydration strategies into your daily routine, you can enhance the effectiveness of your weight loss efforts and experience improved energy levels, better digestion, and a heightened sense of overall vitality. Remember that hydration is a simple yet powerful tool that empowers you to take control of your health and achieve your weight loss goals.

8 Getting Enough Sleep

Getting enough sleep is not just a luxury; it's a crucial factor that significantly impacts various aspects of health, including weight loss. Sleep plays a pivotal role in regulating hormones, metabolism, and appetite, all of which influence weight management. In this chapter, we will explore the importance of quality sleep for weight loss, understand how sleep deprivation affects the body, discuss the connection between sleep and hormones, and provide practical strategies to ensure you prioritize restful sleep on your journey to a healthier you.

The Impact of Sleep on Weight Loss

Hormone Regulation: Sleep influences the balance of hormones that regulate hunger and appetite. Insufficient sleep can disrupt these hormones, leading to increased cravings and overeating.

Metabolism and Energy Expenditure: Adequate sleep supports optimal metabolism and energy expenditure. Sleep deprivation can slow down metabolism and reduce the number of calories burned at rest.

Stress and Emotional Eating: Lack of sleep can contribute to increased stress and emotional eating, which can sabotage weight loss efforts.

Physical Activity: Sleep deprivation may lead to decreased energy levels and motivation, making it harder to engage in regular physical activity.

The Role of Hormones in Sleep and Weight

Leptin and Ghrelin: Leptin is responsible for signaling fullness, while ghrelin stimulates appetite. Sleep deprivation can disrupt the balance of these hormones, leading to increased hunger and reduced satiety.

Cortisol: Sleep deprivation can lead to elevated cortisol levels, a stress hormone linked to weight gain, particularly around the abdominal area.

Insulin Sensitivity: Inadequate sleep can reduce insulin sensitivity, increasing the risk of weight gain and diabetes.

Practical Strategies for Prioritizing Quality Sleep

Establish a Consistent Sleep Schedule:
- Go to bed and wake up at the same time every day, even on weekends.

Consistency helps regulate your body's internal clock.

Create a Relaxing Bedtime Routine:

- Engage in calming activities before bed, such as reading, taking a warm bath, or practicing relaxation techniques like deep breathing.

Limit Screen Time Before Bed:

- The blue light emitted by screens can interfere with the production of melatonin, a hormone that regulates sleep. Avoid screens at least an hour before bedtime.

Optimize Sleep Environment:

- Ensure your bedroom is comfortable, dark, and quiet. Consider using blackout curtains, earplugs, or a white noise machine if needed.

Watch Your Diet:

- Avoid heavy meals, caffeine, and alcohol close to bedtime, as they can disrupt sleep quality.

Stay Active During the Day:

- Engaging in regular physical activity can promote better sleep, but try to finish intense workouts a few hours before bedtime.

Manage Stress:

- Practice stress-reduction techniques such as meditation, yoga, or mindfulness to promote relaxation and improve sleep quality.

Conclusion

Quality sleep is a precious resource that plays an integral role in weight loss and overall well-being. By prioritizing restful sleep, you can regulate hormones, support metabolism, and reduce the risk of overeating and emotional eating. Incorporate practical sleep strategies into your daily routine to create a sleep-conducive environment and establish healthy sleep habits. Remember that sleep is a cornerstone of a healthy lifestyle that empowers you to achieve your weight loss goals and experience improved energy, mental clarity, and emotional resilience.

9 MANAGING STRESS

In the modern world, managing stress is a critical component of achieving successful weight loss and maintaining overall health. Chronic stress can trigger emotional eating, disrupt hormonal balance, and hinder weight loss progress. In this chapter, we will explore the connection between stress and weight gain, understand how stress affects the body, discuss the role of stress in emotional eating, and provide practical strategies to manage stress effectively and support your weight loss journey.

The Stress-Weight Connection

Hormonal Impact: Chronic stress can lead to elevated cortisol levels, which can promote fat storage, particularly around the abdominal area.

Appetite Dysregulation: Stress can disrupt hunger and fullness cues, leading to emotional eating and overconsumption of calorie-dense foods.

Insulin Resistance: Stress can impair insulin sensitivity, affecting blood sugar levels and contributing to weight gain.

Sleep Disruption: Stress can lead to sleep disturbances, which, as discussed in previous chapters, can impact weight loss efforts.

Stress and Emotional Eating

Comfort Food Cravings: Stress often triggers cravings for high-calorie, sugary, or fatty foods as a way to cope with negative emotions.

Mindless Eating: Stress can lead to mindless eating, where you consume food without being fully aware of portion sizes or nutritional choices.

Coping Mechanisms: Emotional eating can provide temporary relief from stress, but it doesn't address the underlying causes of stress.

Practical Strategies for Managing Stress

Mindfulness and Meditation:

- Practice mindfulness meditation to bring your attention to the present moment and reduce stress. Meditation can enhance self-awareness and emotional regulation.

Deep Breathing Exercises:

- Engage in deep breathing exercises to activate the body's relaxation response and reduce stress hormones.

Physical Activity:

- Regular exercise is a natural stress reliever. Engage in activities you enjoy, such as walking, yoga, or dancing, to release endorphins and reduce stress.

Healthy Coping Mechanisms:

- Replace emotional eating with healthier coping mechanisms, such as journaling, talking to a friend, or engaging in a creative activity.

Time Management:

- Create a balanced schedule that includes time for work, relaxation, exercise, and leisure. Avoid overcommitting and prioritize self-care.

Limit Technology Use:

- Set boundaries for screen time to reduce exposure to stress-inducing news or social media.

Seek Support:

- Reach out to friends, family, or a mental health professional for support and guidance in managing stress.

Conclusion

Managing stress is a fundamental aspect of achieving successful weight loss and maintaining a healthy lifestyle. By implementing practical stress management strategies, you can reduce the negative impact of stress on your body, hormones, and eating habits. Remember that stress management is a continuous journey, and building a repertoire of effective coping techniques takes time. By nurturing a balanced and resilient mind, you empower yourself to overcome stress-related challenges and experience improved emotional well-being and overall success on your weight loss journey.

10 TRACKING YOUR PROGRESS

Tracking your progress is a valuable tool that empowers you to achieve successful and sustainable weight loss. It provides insights into your journey, helps you stay accountable, and offers motivation by showcasing your accomplishments. In this chapter, we will explore the importance of tracking progress, understand how it contributes to weight loss success, discuss various methods of tracking, and provide practical tips to make progress tracking an integral part of your weight loss strategy.

The Significance of Tracking Progress

Visibility of Achievements: Tracking your progress allows you to see tangible evidence of your efforts, boosting motivation and confidence.

Accountability: When you track your actions, you're more likely to stay consistent and hold yourself accountable for your choices.

Adjustment and Adaptation: Progress tracking helps you identify what's working and what's not. You can adjust your approach based on real data.

Positive Reinforcement: Celebrating milestones and small victories reinforces positive behavior and encourages continued effort.

Methods of Tracking Progress

Scale: Regular weigh-ins can provide insights into trends and overall progress. However, remember that weight can fluctuate due to various factors, so focus on trends rather than day-to-day changes.

Measurements: Tracking body measurements (such as waist, hips, and arms) can reveal changes in body composition that the scale might not capture.

Photos: Taking before-and-after photos allows you to visually compare your progress over time. Photos can be a powerful source of motivation.

Food Journaling: Recording your meals and snacks can help you become more aware of your eating habits, identify patterns, and make necessary adjustments.

Fitness Tracking Apps: Use apps to log workouts, steps, and activity levels. These apps can provide valuable data for assessing your fitness progress.

Mood and Energy Levels: Tracking your mood, energy levels, and overall well-being can help you connect how your lifestyle choices impact your emotional state.

Practical Tips for Effective Progress Tracking

Set Clear Goals: Define your weight loss goals and what you want to achieve by tracking your progress.

Choose Tracking Methods: Select the tracking methods that align with your goals and preferences.

Establish a Routine: Incorporate progress tracking into your regular routine. Consistency is key to accurate assessment.

Use Technology: Leverage digital tools and apps to simplify and streamline progress tracking.

Document Non-Scale Victories: Celebrate non-scale victories, such as improved energy levels, increased strength, or better sleep.

Reflect and Adjust: Regularly review your tracking data to assess your progress. Adjust your approach based on insights gained.

Stay Positive: Avoid becoming discouraged by occasional setbacks. Remember that progress is not always linear.

Conclusion

Tracking your progress is a dynamic and empowering tool that enhances your weight loss journey. By consistently monitoring your achievements, adjusting your approach, and celebrating your victories, you create a positive feedback loop that keeps you motivated and focused on your goals. Remember that the journey is unique for each individual, and progress tracking helps you discover what works best for you. Embrace the process with patience, commitment, and a growth mindset, and you'll find yourself equipped with the insights and strategies needed to achieve your desired weight loss outcomes and maintain a healthier, happier lifestyle.

11 Building a Support System

Embarking on a weight loss journey can be both exciting and challenging. One of the most valuable assets you can have is a supportive network of friends, family, and like-minded individuals who encourage and motivate you along the way. In this chapter, we will explore the importance of building a support system for weight loss, understand how it contributes to success, discuss the types of support available, and provide practical strategies for cultivating a strong and effective support network.

The Impact of Support Systems on Weight Loss

> Motivation and Accountability: A support system provides motivation, encouragement, and accountability, helping you stay focused on your goals.

> Shared Experiences: Connecting with others who are on similar journeys fosters a sense of belonging and shared experiences.

> Emotional Support: A support network offers a safe space to discuss challenges, setbacks, and emotions related to weight loss.

Positive Influence: Surrounding yourself with individuals who prioritize health and well-being can positively influence your choices and habits.

Types of Support Systems

Personal Network:
- Friends, family members, and colleagues who support your goals and offer encouragement.

Online Communities:
- Social media groups, forums, and online platforms where individuals share their experiences, challenges, and successes.

Weight Loss Groups:
- Joining a local or virtual weight loss group provides opportunities to connect with like-minded individuals, attend meetings, and share strategies.

Professional Support:
- Working with a registered dietitian, personal trainer, or therapist can provide personalized guidance and expertise.

Practical Strategies for Building a Support System

Communicate Your Goals:

- Share your weight loss goals with your personal network, explaining why they are important to you.

Set Expectations:

- Clearly communicate the type of support you need, whether it's encouragement, accountability, or understanding.

Engage in Online Communities:

- Participate in online forums, social media groups, and platforms dedicated to weight loss and healthy living.

Attend Support Groups:

- Join local weight loss or fitness groups to connect with individuals who share similar goals.

Choose Positive Influences:

- Surround yourself with individuals who uplift and encourage you, avoiding negativity or unsupportive attitudes.

Seek Professional Guidance:

- Work with professionals who can provide expert advice tailored to your needs.

Reciprocate Support:

- Offer support to others within your network, creating a mutually beneficial environment.

Conclusion

Building a support system is an essential aspect of achieving successful weight loss and maintaining a healthy lifestyle. By cultivating a network of individuals who uplift, motivate, and understand your journey, you create a foundation for long-term success. Remember that support can come from various sources, both personal and virtual. Whether it's through friends, family, online communities, or professionals, the presence of a supportive network can make all the difference in your ability to overcome challenges, stay focused on your goals, and celebrate your achievements. Embrace the power of connection, give and receive support with an open heart, and discover the strength and resilience that come from being part of a supportive community.